THE COMPLETE ANTI-INFLAMMATORY DIET COOKBOOK FOR BEGINNERS

Discover Easy and Flavorful Recipes to Boost Your Immune System and Effectively Reduce Inflammation for Optimal Wellness and Health

Bonus: 30-day Meal Plan for Mediterranean diet

By Vanessa R. Haddock

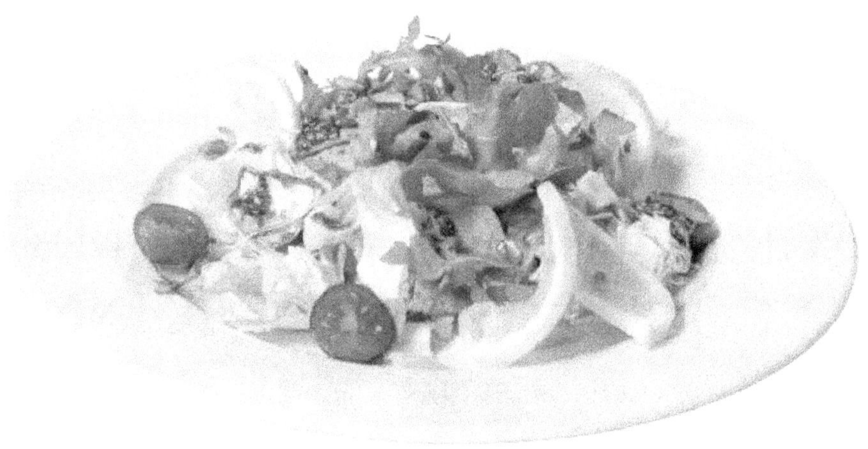

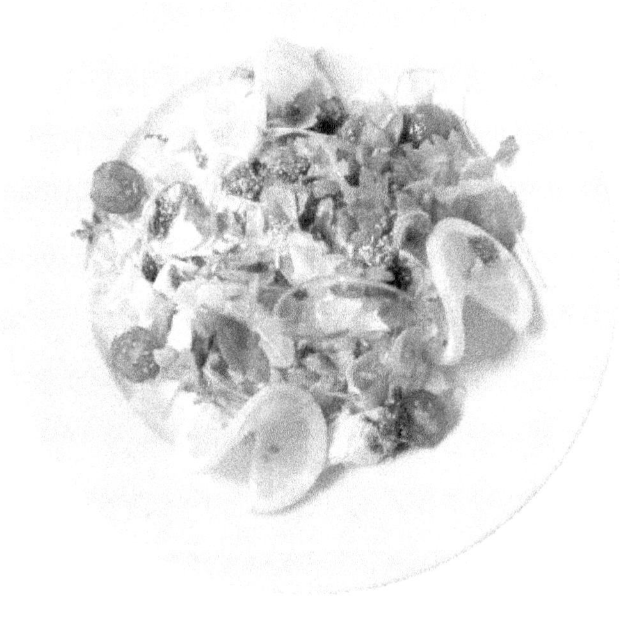

Copyright

Disclaimer

The information provided in this book is for general informational purposes only. While every effort has been made to ensure the accuracy and completeness of the content, the author makes no representations or warranties of any kind, express or implied, about the completeness, accuracy, reliability, suitability, or availability concerning the information, products, services, or related graphics contained in this book.

Any reliance you place on such information is strictly at your own risk. The author will not be liable for any losses or damages arising from the use of this book.

Furthermore, this book is not intended to provide medical, nutritional, or professional advice. Readers are encouraged to consult with qualified professionals for advice specific to their individual circumstances.

The inclusion of certain products, brands, or services in this book does not constitute an endorsement or recommendation. The author does not have any financial interests or affiliations with these entities.

Every effort is made to respect copyright laws and regulations. If you believe that any content in this book infringes upon your copyright, please contact the author immediately.

The author reserves the right to make changes to the content of this book at any time, without prior notice.

HERE IS YOUR 30-DAYS MEAL PLAN BONUS

All recipes are discussed in the book

Day 1:

- Breakfast: Kale and Spinach Smoothie
- Lunch: Roasted Vegetable Wrap
- Dinner: Eggplant Rollatini with Tomato Sauce

Day 2:

- Breakfast: Quinoa Breakfast Bowl
- Lunch: Greek Salmon Salad
- Dinner: Lemon Dill Baked Cod

Day 3:

- Breakfast: Broccoli and Parmesan Cheese Omelet
- Lunch: Shrimp and Quinoa Stir-Fry
- Dinner: Buffalo Cauliflower Tacos

Day 4:

- Breakfast: Avocado and Arugula Omelet
- Lunch: Couscous and Chickpea Salad
- Dinner: Chicken Cali Soup

Day 5:

- Breakfast: Waffles with Feta and Smoked Salmon
- Lunch: Teriyaki Tofu Rice
- Dinner: Butternut Squash and Sage Risotto

Day 6:

- Breakfast: Egg Salad Avocado Toast
- Lunch: Avocado Chicken Salad
- Dinner: Cauliflower Steak with Pesto

Day 7:

- Breakfast: Strawberry and Yoghurt Parfait
- Lunch: Spicy Ramen Cup of Noodles
- Dinner: Vegetarian Stuffed Bell Peppers

Day 8:

- Breakfast: Granola Breakfast Protein Balls
- Lunch: Chicken Tuna Salad
- Dinner: Portobello Mushroom Bell

Day 9:

- Breakfast: Chia Seed Pudding Parfait
- Lunch: Sweet Potato and Lentil Stew
- Dinner: Minestra Maritata

Day 10:

- Breakfast: Cacao Berry Smoothie
- Lunch: Turmeric Chicken Wrap
- Dinner: Sheet Pan Shrimp and Beets

Day 11:

- Breakfast: Spinach and Feta Scrambled Egg Pitas
- Lunch: Roasted Vegetable Wrap
- Dinner: Lemon Dill Baked Cod

Day 12:

- Breakfast: Kale and Spinach Smoothie
- Lunch: Avocado Chicken Salad
- Dinner: Vegetarian Stuffed Bell Peppers

Day 13:

- Breakfast: Egg and Veggie Muffin Cups
- Lunch: Couscous and Chickpea Salad
- Dinner: Cauliflower Steak with Pesto

Day 14:

- Breakfast: Avocado and Arugula Omelet
- Lunch: Greek Salmon Salad
- Dinner: Butternut Squash and Sage Risotto

Day 15:

- Breakfast: Waffles with Feta and Smoked Salmon
- Lunch: Teriyaki Tofu Rice
- Dinner: Eggplant Rollatini with Tomato Sauce

Day 16:

- Breakfast: Egg Salad Avocado Toast
- Lunch: Spicy Ramen Cup of Noodles
- Dinner: Buffalo Cauliflower Tacos

Day 17:

- Breakfast: Quinoa Breakfast Bowl
- Lunch: Roasted Vegetable Wrap
- Dinner: Chicken Cali Soup

Day 18:

- Breakfast: Strawberry and Yoghurt Parfait
- Lunch: Couscous and Chickpea Salad
- Dinner: Portobello Mushroom Bell

Day 19:

- Breakfast: Granola Breakfast Protein Balls
- Lunch: Avocado Chicken Salad
- Dinner: Sheet Pan Shrimp and Beets

Day 20:

- Breakfast: Chia Seed Pudding Parfait
- Lunch: Sweet Potato and Lentil Stew
- Dinner: Minestra Maritata

Day 21:

- Breakfast: Cacao Berry Smoothie
- Lunch: Turmeric Chicken Wrap
- Dinner: Lemon Dill Baked Cod

Day 22:

- Breakfast: Spinach and Feta Scrambled Egg Pitas
- Lunch: Teriyaki Tofu Rice
- Dinner: Butternut Squash and Sage Risotto

Day 23:

- ➢ Breakfast: Avocado and Arugula Omelet
- ➢ Lunch: Greek Salmon Salad
- ➢ Dinner: Cauliflower Steak with Pesto

Day 24:

- ➢ Breakfast: Egg and Veggie Muffin Cups
- ➢ Lunch: Roasted Vegetable Wrap
- ➢ Dinner: Vegetarian Stuffed Bell Peppers

Day 25:

- ➢ Breakfast: Waffles with Feta and Smoked Salmon
- ➢ Lunch: Avocado Chicken Salad
- ➢ Dinner: Sheet Pan Shrimp and Beets

Day 26:

- ➢ Breakfast: Strawberry and Yoghurt Parfait
- ➢ Lunch: Spicy Ramen Cup of Noodles
- ➢ Dinner: Buffalo Cauliflower Tacos

Day 27:

- ➢ Breakfast: Quinoa Breakfast Bowl
- ➢ Lunch: Couscous and Chickpea Salad
- ➢ Dinner: Eggplant Rollatini with Tomato Sauce

Day 28:

- ➢ Breakfast: Granola Breakfast Protein Balls
- ➢ Lunch: Chicken Tuna Salad
- ➢ Dinner: Portobello Mushroom Bell

Day 29:

- ➢ Breakfast: Chia Seed Pudding Parfait
- ➢ Lunch: Sweet Potato and Lentil Stew
- ➢ Dinner: Minestra Maritata

Day 30:

- ➢ Breakfast: Cacao Berry Smoothie
- ➢ Lunch: Turmeric Chicken Wrap
- ➢ Dinner: Lemon Dill Baked Cod

About the Author

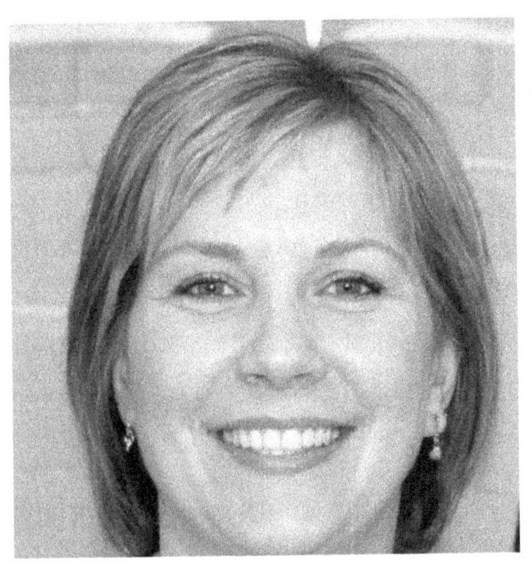

Vanessa R. Haddock is not just a name; it's a culinary journey, a tale of flavors woven into the fabric of a life dedicated to the art of gastronomy. A seasoned chef with a passion for healthy living and an advocate for a balanced lifestyle, Vanessa's story is a symphony of taste, nutrition, and well-being.

Vanessa's culinary odyssey began in the bustling kitchens of renowned establishments, where she honed her skills and developed an insatiable curiosity for the endless possibilities that food offers. Her journey took her from mastering classic techniques to embracing innovative approaches, always with the goal of creating dishes that not only delight the palate but also nurture the body.

The roots of Vanessa's culinary philosophy lie in her belief that food is not just sustenance; it is an experience. It is a medium through which we connect with our senses, with each other, and with the world around us. This philosophy is at the heart of Vanessa's culinary creations, where she artfully combines fresh, seasonal ingredients to produce dishes that are as visually appealing as they are delicious.

As a chef deeply committed to healthy eating, Vanessa understands the profound impact that food choices have on our well-being. Her exploration of nutrition goes beyond the kitchen, leading her to advocate for a holistic approach to health. Vanessa sees food as more than just fuel; it's a source of nourishment for the body, mind, and soul.

Her dedication to this holistic perspective is not just professional; it's a personal commitment to living a life in harmony with nature's bounty.

Beyond the tantalizing aromas and exquisite tastes, Vanessa's journey extends to the intimate sphere of her personal life. Married and deeply in love, Vanessa's relationship provides the foundation for the warmth and care she infuses into her culinary creations. The joy and fulfillment she experiences in her personal life become the secret ingredients that elevate her dishes, turning them into more than just meals—they are expressions of love, connection, and shared moments around the table.

Vanessa's culinary prowess is not confined to the professional kitchen; it extends to the community. As an advocate for healthy living, she engages in outreach programs, cooking classes, and educational initiatives, sharing her knowledge and passion with a wider audience. Her goal is to inspire others to embrace a lifestyle that prioritizes wellness without compromising on the pleasure of eating.

In the pages of her cookbook, Vanessa invites you to join her on this multifaceted journey. It's not just a collection of recipes; it's a narrative of a life steeped in the love of food, a journey that intertwines the sensory joys of cooking with the profound understanding that what we eat shapes not only our bodies but our entire experience of life.

So, as you turn the pages of Vanessa R. Haddock's culinary chronicle, be prepared to embark on a voyage that transcends the kitchen. It's an exploration of taste, a celebration of health, and an invitation to savor the richness of life with every delectable bite.

Table of content

Introduction

Welcome to "The Complete Anti-Inflammatory Diet Cookbook for Beginners," a comprehensive guide designed to empower you on your journey toward a healthier, more vibrant life. In today's fast-paced world, prioritizing our well-being is of utmost importance, and understanding the impact of our dietary choices on inflammation can be a pivotal step towards achieving optimal health.

Inflammation, while a natural and necessary process for healing, can become problematic when it persists chronically. This cookbook is crafted to introduce you to the transformative potential of an anti-inflammatory diet, a lifestyle approach that harnesses the healing properties of wholesome, nutrient-dense foods.

The journey begins by unraveling the fundamentals of inflammation, providing insights into its role within the body and the far-reaching consequences of chronic inflammation on overall health. As we delve into the foundational aspects of an anti-inflammatory diet, you'll discover the wealth of nutrients present in vibrant fruits, vegetables, lean proteins, and nourishing herbs and spices.

With practical advice on meal planning and essential kitchen tools, this cookbook guides you through crafting balanced and flavorful meals. From energizing breakfast choices to satisfying lunches and wholesome dinners, each chapter is curated to inspire creativity in the kitchen while prioritizing your well-being.

Snacking smartly and indulging in desserts with a purpose are explored in dedicated chapters, proving that enjoying tasty treats can align seamlessly with an anti-inflammatory lifestyle. Discover the art of making healthy snacks and desserts that not only satisfy your taste buds but also contribute positively to your overall health.

Recognizing that conscious eating extends beyond what we include in our diets, a specific chapter highlights foods to avoid that may contribute to inflammation. This crucial section empowers you with knowledge, enabling you to make informed choices that align with your health goals.

Building a sustainable anti-inflammatory lifestyle goes beyond the kitchen, and our guide provides insights into maintaining consistency and overcoming challenges. Staying motivated on your journey is key, and this section offers practical tips to integrate these principles into your daily life.

"The Complete Anti-Inflammatory Diet Cookbook for Beginners" invites you to embark on a culinary adventure that prioritizes health without compromising on flavor. Whether you are a seasoned cook or stepping into the kitchen for the first time, this cookbook is your companion in creating nourishing, delicious meals that support your journey to optimal health.

Let the pages that follow be a source of inspiration, education, and empowerment as you embrace the transformative potential of an anti-inflammatory lifestyle.

Your journey to a healthier, more vibrant you starts here.

Understanding Inflammation

The Basics of Inflammation

Inflammation is a fundamental and complex biological response that our bodies employ to protect and heal. When our immune system detects injury, infection, or harmful stimuli, it initiates a cascade of events to eliminate the threat and restore tissue integrity. This intricate process involves a coordinated interplay of cells, proteins, and signaling molecules, creating what is commonly known as the inflammatory response.

<u>The Process Unveiled:</u>

➢ **Initiation:**

Inflammation typically begins with the recognition of harmful stimuli, such as pathogens, damaged cells, or irritants. Immune cells, primarily white blood cells, release signaling molecules like cytokines, signaling the alarm and initiating the response.

➢ **Dilation of Blood Vessels:**

Blood vessels near the affected area dilate to increase blood flow, allowing immune cells to reach the site more efficiently. This results in warmth and redness, classic signs of inflammation.

➢ **Increased Permeability:**

The walls of blood vessels become more permeable, facilitating the movement of immune cells, proteins, and nutrients to the site of injury or infection. Swelling, another hallmark of inflammation, occurs as fluid accumulates in the tissues.

> **Migration of Immune Cells:**

White blood cells, including neutrophils and macrophages, migrate to the affected area. These cells are tasked with engulfing and neutralizing pathogens, removing damaged cells, and promoting tissue repair.

> **Tissue Repair and Healing:**

Once the threat is eliminated, anti-inflammatory signals help resolve the response. Specialized cells, such as fibroblasts, aid in tissue repair, ensuring the restoration of normal function and structure.

TYPES OF INFLAMMATION:

Inflammation can be classified into two types: acute and chronic.

1. **Acute Inflammation:** This is a rapid and self-limiting response that occurs in response to injury or infection. It is a crucial defense mechanism that helps the body eliminate the source of harm and initiate the healing process.
2. **Chronic Inflammation:** Unlike acute inflammation, chronic inflammation is persistent and can last for weeks, months, or even years. It is often low-grade and may not produce the classic signs of redness and swelling. Chronic inflammation is associated with a range of health conditions, including autoimmune diseases, metabolic disorders, and certain cancers.

Impact of Chronic Inflammation on Health

Inflammation, when functioning as a temporary and controlled response, is a crucial aspect of the body's defense and healing mechanisms. However, when inflammation becomes chronic, persisting over an extended period, it can lead to a cascade of detrimental effects on overall health. Chronic inflammation has been implicated as a contributing factor in the development and progression of various diseases, affecting virtually every organ system in the body.

1. Cardiovascular Health:

Chronic inflammation plays a pivotal role in the development of cardiovascular diseases. The persistent inflammatory response can damage blood vessels, contributing to the formation of atherosclerosis (hardening of the arteries) and increasing the risk of heart attacks and strokes.

2. Metabolic Disorders:

Conditions such as obesity and type 2 diabetes are closely linked to chronic inflammation. Inflammation can interfere with the body's ability to regulate insulin, leading to insulin resistance. This, in turn, contributes to elevated blood sugar levels and an increased risk of developing diabetes.

3. Autoimmune Diseases:

Chronic inflammation is a hallmark of autoimmune diseases, where the immune system mistakenly attacks the body's own tissues. Conditions such as rheumatoid arthritis, lupus, and inflammatory bowel diseases are examples of autoimmune disorders driven by persistent inflammation.

4. Neurological Disorders:

The impact of chronic inflammation extends to the nervous system, contributing to neurodegenerative diseases like Alzheimer's and Parkinson's. Inflammation in the brain can disrupt normal cellular function and contribute to the progression of these debilitating conditions.

5. Respiratory Conditions:

Chronic inflammation is a common feature in respiratory disorders such as chronic obstructive pulmonary disease (COPD) and asthma. Inflammatory responses in the airways can lead to breathing difficulties and exacerbate symptoms in individuals with pre-existing respiratory conditions.

6. Cancer Risk:

While chronic inflammation itself is not a direct cause of cancer, it creates an environment conducive to the initiation and progression of cancer cells. Persistent inflammation can lead to DNA damage, impaired immune responses, and the promotion of tumor growth.

7. Joint Health:

Conditions like osteoarthritis and rheumatoid arthritis involve chronic inflammation affecting the joints. Inflammatory processes contribute to the degradation of cartilage, leading to pain, stiffness, and reduced joint function.

8. Gastrointestinal Disorders:

Chronic inflammation can contribute to gastrointestinal issues, including inflammatory bowel diseases like Crohn's disease and ulcerative colitis. Inflammation in the digestive tract can lead to symptoms such as abdominal pain, diarrhea, and malabsorption of nutrients.

Understanding the impact of chronic inflammation underscores the importance of adopting lifestyle practices that promote a balanced immune response. An anti-inflammatory diet, regular physical activity, stress management, and adequate sleep are essential components of a holistic approach to mitigate chronic inflammation and support overall health.

By recognizing the role of chronic inflammation in various health conditions, individuals can take proactive steps toward preventive healthcare, making informed choices that contribute to a healthier, more resilient body.

Benefits of Adopting an Anti-Inflammatory Diet

Embracing an anti-inflammatory diet isn't just a culinary choice; it's a transformative lifestyle approach with far-reaching benefits for overall health and well-being. By making mindful choices in your dietary habits, you empower your body to manage inflammation effectively, and the positive effects extend across various aspects of your physical and mental health.

1. Reduction of Chronic Inflammation:

The primary objective of an anti-inflammatory diet is to mitigate chronic inflammation, the root cause of many health issues. By incorporating foods rich in anti-inflammatory properties, you create an environment in which your body can better regulate the inflammatory response, reducing the risk of chronic diseases.

2. Cardiovascular Health Improvement:

Adopting an anti-inflammatory diet can positively impact cardiovascular health. By focusing on nutrient-dense, whole foods, you support healthy blood vessels, reduce the risk of atherosclerosis, and promote optimal heart function. This can contribute to a lower risk of heart attacks, strokes, and other cardiovascular diseases.

3. Weight Management Support:

Many anti-inflammatory foods are naturally low in calories and high in fiber, aiding in weight management. Maintaining a healthy weight is crucial for reducing inflammation, as excess body fat can contribute to chronic low-grade inflammation. The diet's emphasis on nutrient-rich options helps support sustainable weight loss or maintenance.

4. Improved Blood Sugar Control:

An anti-inflammatory diet, particularly one that focuses on whole grains, lean proteins, and colorful vegetables, can assist in stabilizing blood sugar levels. This is especially beneficial for individuals at risk of or managing type 2 diabetes, as it helps prevent insulin resistance and supports overall metabolic health.

5. Enhanced Joint Health:

Anti-inflammatory foods rich in omega-3 fatty acids, antioxidants, and other beneficial compounds can contribute to improved joint health. This is particularly beneficial for individuals dealing with conditions like arthritis, as the diet may help reduce inflammation and alleviate symptoms.

6. Support for Cognitive Function:

The brain benefits from an anti-inflammatory diet that includes omega-3 fatty acids and antioxidants. These nutrients have been associated with improved cognitive function, reduced risk of neurodegenerative diseases, and better mental well-being.

7. Digestive Wellness:

An anti-inflammatory diet that prioritizes fiber-rich foods and gut-friendly options promotes a healthy digestive system. It can help prevent or manage gastrointestinal issues, such as inflammatory bowel diseases, by supporting the balance of gut microbiota.

8. Boosted Immune System:

Nutrient-dense foods inherent in an anti-inflammatory diet provide essential vitamins, minerals, and antioxidants crucial for a robust immune system. By supporting immune function, you enhance your body's ability to defend against infections and illnesses.

9. Balanced Hormones:

Certain foods in an anti-inflammatory diet, such as those rich in omega-3 fatty acids and antioxidants, can contribute to hormonal balance. This can be particularly beneficial for women dealing with conditions like polycystic ovary syndrome (PCOS) or those experiencing hormonal fluctuations.

10. Increased Energy and Vitality:

Adopting an anti-inflammatory diet can lead to increased energy levels and a sense of vitality. Nutrient-dense foods provide the necessary fuel for the body's functions, helping to combat fatigue and support overall well-being.

In conclusion, the benefits of embracing an anti-inflammatory diet extend beyond the plate. By making thoughtful and health-conscious choices in your dietary patterns, you cultivate an environment within your body that promotes longevity, resilience, and a higher quality of life.

Foundation of an Anti-Inflammatory Diet

Nutrient-Rich Foods

Powerhouse Fruits and Vegetables

The cornerstone of an anti-inflammatory diet lies in the vibrant colors of fruits and vegetables. Rich in antioxidants, such as vitamins A, C, and E, as well as phytonutrients like flavonoids and carotenoids, these foods combat oxidative stress and inflammation. Incorporating a rainbow of produce into your meals ensures a broad spectrum of health-promoting compounds.

Whole Grains and Fiber

Whole grains, such as quinoa, brown rice, oats, and whole wheat, are integral to an anti-inflammatory diet. They provide a rich source of fiber, which not only supports digestive health but also helps regulate blood sugar levels. The complex carbohydrates found in whole grains release energy gradually, promoting sustained vitality.

Healthy Fats

Omega-3 and Beyond Healthy fats, particularly those high in omega-3 fatty acids, play a crucial role in reducing inflammation. Foods like fatty fish (salmon, mackerel), flaxseeds, chia seeds, and walnuts are excellent sources of omega-3s. These fats contribute to the production of anti-inflammatory compounds in the body, helping to balance the inflammatory response.

Lean Proteins

Lean protein sources, including poultry, fish, legumes, and tofu, form an essential component of an anti-inflammatory diet. Protein is vital for tissue repair, immune function, and maintaining muscle mass. Choosing lean, plant-based, or fatty fish options ensures a balance of amino acids without an excess of saturated fats.

Herbs and Spices

Herbs and spices not only add flavor to dishes but also offer potent anti-inflammatory properties. Turmeric, ginger, garlic, cinnamon, and rosemary are renowned for their ability to reduce inflammation and oxidative stress. Incorporating these flavorful elements into your meals enhances both taste and nutritional value.

Nuts and Seeds

Nuts and seeds, such as almonds, walnuts, chia seeds, and flaxseeds, are rich in healthy fats, fiber, and antioxidants. They make for satisfying snacks and additions to meals, providing a nutrient-dense boost that supports heart health and helps regulate inflammation.

Limiting Processed Foods

While emphasizing nutrient-rich foods, an anti-inflammatory diet encourages the reduction of processed and refined foods. These often contain additives, preservatives, and unhealthy fats that can contribute to inflammation. Choosing whole, unprocessed foods promotes a cleaner, more health-supportive eating pattern.

In essence, the foundation of an anti-inflammatory diet lies in embracing a variety of nutrient-dense foods that work synergistically to create an internal environment conducive to health and vitality. By prioritizing these whole foods, you empower your body to thrive and naturally combat chronic inflammation.

Foods to Avoid for an Anti-Inflammatory Diet

In conjunction with emphasizing nutrient-rich foods, adopting an anti-inflammatory diet involves being mindful of choices that can contribute to inflammation. Limiting or avoiding certain foods known for their pro-inflammatory properties is essential to support the goal of reducing chronic inflammation and promoting overall well-being.

> **Processed and Refined Sugars:**

High levels of added sugars, commonly found in sugary beverages, candies, pastries, and many processed foods, can contribute to inflammation. These sugars may lead to increased insulin resistance and oxidative stress, both linked to inflammatory processes.

> **Saturated and Trans Fats:**

Foods high in saturated and trans fats, such as fried foods, processed snacks, and certain margarines, can promote inflammation. These fats may activate inflammatory pathways and contribute to the development of cardiovascular diseases.

> **Processed and Red Meats:**

Processed meats, including sausages, hot dogs, and certain deli meats, contain preservatives and additives that can trigger inflammation. Red meats, particularly when processed or overcooked, may produce compounds linked to inflammatory responses.

> **Refined Carbohydrates:**

Refined carbohydrates, like those found in white bread, white rice, and sugary cereals, can cause spikes in blood sugar levels. Elevated blood sugar levels may contribute to insulin resistance and chronic inflammation.

➢ Excessive Omega-6 Fatty Acids:

While omega-6 fatty acids are essential, an imbalance with omega-3 fatty acids can contribute to inflammation. Foods high in omega-6, such as certain vegetable oils (soybean, corn, and sunflower oil), should be consumed in moderation to maintain a healthy ratio.

➢ Artificial Additives and Sweeteners:

Processed foods containing artificial additives, preservatives, and sweeteners may trigger inflammatory responses in some individuals. Opting for whole, minimally processed foods helps avoid exposure to these potential inflammatory agents.

➢ Highly Processed and Fried Foods:

Highly processed and fried foods often contain unhealthy fats, high levels of sodium, and various additives. These can contribute to inflammation and may have negative effects on overall health when consumed regularly.

➢ High Sodium Foods:

Excessive sodium intake, often found in processed and packaged foods, can contribute to water retention and may promote inflammation. Monitoring and reducing sodium consumption can support overall cardiovascular health.

➢ Alcohol:

While moderate alcohol consumption may have certain health benefits, excessive or chronic alcohol intake can lead to inflammation and damage various organs, including the liver. Limiting alcohol intake aligns with the principles of an anti-inflammatory lifestyle.

➢ Highly Processed Vegetable Oils:

Certain vegetable oils, like soybean and corn oil, which are high in omega-6 fatty acids can contribute to an imbalance in the omega-3 to omega-6 ratio. Choosing oils rich in monounsaturated fats, such as olive oil, may be a healthier alternative.

Getting Started

Setting Your Health Goals

Embarking on the journey of adopting an anti-inflammatory diet is an empowering step towards enhancing your overall health and well-being. Setting clear and achievable health goals provides a roadmap for your wellness journey, helping you stay focused, motivated, and committed to positive changes. **Here's a guide to help you set effective health goals within the context of an anti-inflammatory lifestyle:**

1. Define Specific Objectives:

Clearly outline your health objectives, ensuring they are specific, measurable, achievable, relevant, and time-bound (SMART). For example, instead of a vague goal like "eat healthier," specify "consume at least five servings of colorful vegetables daily for the next four weeks."

2. Identify Personal Motivations:

Understand your personal motivations for adopting an anti-inflammatory diet. Whether it's reducing inflammation, improving energy levels, or managing a specific health condition, knowing your "why" can strengthen your commitment to your goals.

3. Start Gradually:

Introduce changes gradually to make the transition to an anti-inflammatory lifestyle more sustainable. Setting smaller, achievable goals initially allows you to build momentum and adapt to new dietary habits without feeling overwhelmed.

4. Focus on Balanced Nutrition:

Ensure your health goals prioritize a balanced intake of nutrients. Set goals related to incorporating a variety of colorful fruits and vegetables, choosing whole grains, incorporating lean proteins, and optimizing healthy fats. Strive for a well-rounded and nourishing diet.

5. Meal Planning and Preparation:

Establish goals related to meal planning and preparation. This may include setting aside time each week to plan meals, preparing a grocery list focused on anti-inflammatory foods, and dedicating time for batch cooking to streamline healthy eating.

6. Hydration Goals:

Include hydration in your health goals. Set specific targets for daily water intake, aiming for at least eight glasses a day. Staying well-hydrated is crucial for supporting bodily functions and maintaining overall health.

7. Incorporate Physical Activity:

Recognize the importance of physical activity in an anti-inflammatory lifestyle. Set goals related to regular exercise, whether it's incorporating daily walks, engaging in strength training, or practicing yoga. Physical activity complements dietary efforts in promoting overall health.

8. Manage Stress:

Recognize the impact of stress on inflammation and overall health. Set goals related to stress management, incorporating practices such as mindfulness, meditation, or deep breathing exercises into your daily routine.

Remember that each person's journey to better health is unique. Tailor your goals to align with your personal preferences, lifestyle, and health status. Regularly reassess and adjust your goals as needed to ensure they remain challenging yet achievable, fostering a sustainable and fulfilling anti-inflammatory lifestyle.

Essential Kitchen Tools

Equipping your kitchen with the right tools can streamline your efforts in preparing nourishing, anti-inflammatory meals. **Here's a list of essential kitchen tools to help you embrace a health-conscious culinary lifestyle:**

1. Quality Knives:

Invest in a set of sharp, high-quality knives for chopping, slicing, and dicing fruits, vegetables, and proteins. A chef's knife, paring knife, and serrated knife can cover a range of cutting needs.

2. Cutting Boards:

Choose durable and easy-to-clean cutting boards, preferably in different colors to designate specific boards for various food groups (e.g., one for vegetables, one for meats). This helps prevent cross-contamination.

3. Blender or Food Processor:

A blender or food processor is invaluable for creating smoothies, soups, sauces, and dressings. These appliances make it easy to incorporate nutrient-rich ingredients like fruits, vegetables, and nuts into your diet.

4. Vegetable Spiralizer:

A spiralizer allows you to turn vegetables like zucchini, carrots, or sweet potatoes into noodle-like strands. This versatile tool adds variety to your meals and facilitates the incorporation of more vegetables.

5. Citrus Juicer:

Extracting fresh juice from citrus fruits like lemons and limes is a breeze with a citrus juicer. Fresh citrus juice is a flavorful addition to dressings, marinades, and beverages.

6. Microplane Grater:

A microplane grater is ideal for finely grating ingredients like ginger, garlic, or citrus zest. It enhances the flavors in your dishes without the need for large quantities.

7. Steamer Basket:

A steamer basket is a simple yet effective tool for gently cooking vegetables while preserving their nutrients. Steaming is a healthy cooking method that supports an anti-inflammatory diet.

8. Non-Stick Pans and Pots:

Non-stick cookware reduces the need for excessive oil and makes cooking and cleaning easier. Opt for high-quality pans and pots with a non-toxic coating.

9. Baking Sheets and Pans:

Baking sheets and pans are versatile for roasting vegetables, preparing sheet pan meals, and baking healthy treats. Choose those made from durable materials like stainless steel or cast iron.

10. Mason Jars or Glass Containers:

Mason jars or glass containers are excellent for storing batch-cooked meals, salads, and homemade sauces. They are convenient, eco-friendly, and keep your food fresh.

11. Digital Kitchen Scale:

A digital kitchen scale ensures accurate measurements, especially when following recipes for an anti-inflammatory diet that may require precise ingredient quantities.

12. Herb and Spice Grinder:

Freshly ground herbs and spices enhance the flavor of your dishes. A dedicated grinder allows you to maximize the potency of anti-inflammatory spices like turmeric, ginger, and black pepper.

13. Measuring Cups and Spoons:

Accurate measurements are crucial in cooking. Having a set of measuring cups and spoons ensures precision when portioning ingredients for your anti-inflammatory recipes.

14. Salad Spinner:

A salad spinner makes it easy to wash and dry leafy greens thoroughly. Crisp and dry greens are ideal for creating vibrant salads.

15. Kitchen Timer:

A reliable kitchen timer helps you keep track of cooking times, ensuring that your meals are perfectly cooked without overcooking or undercooking.

By incorporating these essential kitchen tools into your culinary space, you'll be well-equipped to embark on a seamless and enjoyable journey towards adopting an anti-inflammatory diet.

Stocking Anti-Inflammatory Pantry Staples

Building a well-stocked pantry with anti-inflammatory staples lays the foundation for creating nutritious and flavorful meals that support your health goals. **Here's a comprehensive list to guide you in filling your pantry with ingredients that align with an anti-inflammatory diet:**

1. Whole Grains:
- Brown rice
- Quinoa
- Oats
- Bulgur
- Farro
- Whole wheat pasta

2 Legumes:
- Lentils
- Chickpeas
- Black beans
- Kidney beans
- Cannellini beans

3. Healthy Fats:

- Extra virgin olive oil
- Avocado oil
- Nuts (almonds, walnuts)
- Seeds (flaxseeds, chia seeds)
- Nut butters (almond, peanut, cashew)

4. Canned Tomatoes:

- Whole tomatoes
- Diced tomatoes
- Tomato sauce (without added sugars)

5. Herbs and Spices:

- Turmeric
- Ginger
- Garlic
- Cinnamon
- Rosemary
- Thyme
- Basil
- Cumin
- Coriander
- Paprika
- Black pepper

6. Whole Herbs:

- Fresh basil
- Fresh cilantro
- Fresh parsley
- Fresh mint

7. Vinegars:

- Apple cider vinegar
- Balsamic vinegar

8. Whole Grains and Seeds:

- Flaxseeds
- Chia seeds
- Hemp seeds
- Sunflower seeds

9. Canned Fish:

- Salmon
- Sardines
- Mackerel

10. Whole Grains and Flour Alternatives:

- Almond flour
- Coconut flour
- Whole wheat flour
- Oat flour

11. Non-Dairy Milk Alternatives:

- Almond milk
- Coconut milk
- Oat milk

12. Sweeteners:

- Honey (raw, unpasteurized)
- Maple syrup
- Stevia

13. Broths and Stocks:

- Low-sodium vegetable broth
- Low-sodium chicken broth
- Bone broth

4. Canned Legumes:

- Cannellini beans
- Chickpeas
- Black beans
- Kidney beans

15. Whole Grain Snacks:

- Brown rice cakes
- Whole grain crackers
- Popcorn kernels

16. Non-Dairy Yogurt:

- Almond yogurt
- Coconut yogurt

18. Condiments:

- Mustard
- Tahini
- Hummus

19. Gluten-Free Grains:

- Quinoa
- Brown rice
- Millet

20. Teas:

- Green tea
- Turmeric tea
- Ginger tea

By keeping these anti-inflammatory pantry staples on hand, you'll have a solid base for preparing a variety of nutrient-rich and delicious meals that support your overall health and well-being. Regularly check and replenish your pantry items to ensure you can create anti-inflammatory dishes whenever the inspiration strikes.

Meal Planning Tips for Success

Meal planning is a key component of maintaining a successful and sustainable anti-inflammatory diet. **Here are five tips to help you streamline your meal planning process and set yourself up for success:**

1. Set Realistic Goals:

Begin with realistic and achievable meal planning goals. Start with planning for a few days or a week, and gradually extend to longer periods as you become more comfortable with the process. Consider your schedule, cooking skills, and preferences when setting your goals.

2. Create a Weekly Schedule:

Develop a weekly meal schedule that includes breakfast, lunch, dinner, and snacks. Having a structured plan reduces the temptation to opt for convenient yet less healthy food choices. Plan meals that are diverse, incorporating a variety of anti-inflammatory foods.

3. Batch Cooking and Prep:

Embrace batch cooking and meal preparation to save time on busy weekdays. Cook larger quantities of staples like grains, proteins, and vegetables, and store them in portion-sized containers. Prepping ingredients in advance can significantly speed up the cooking process during the week.

4. Plan Balanced and Colorful Meals:

Prioritize balanced and colorful meals to ensure a wide range of nutrients. Incorporate a variety of fruits, vegetables, whole grains, lean proteins, and healthy fats into each meal. Aim for a diverse array of colors on your plate, as different colors often signify different beneficial compounds.

5. **Stay Flexible and Rotate Recipes:**

Be flexible with your meal plan to accommodate unexpected changes in your schedule or preferences. Have a list of go-to recipes that are quick and easy for those hectic days. Rotate your recipes to maintain variety and prevent culinary boredom, keeping your meals exciting and enjoyable.

Bonus Tip: Use a Meal Planning Template:

> ➤ Consider using a meal planning template or app to organize your weekly meals. This can help you visualize your plan, track your grocery needs, and stay on top of your anti-inflammatory dietary goals. Having a structured format makes it easier to stick to your plan and fosters consistency.

Meal planning not only supports your anti-inflammatory diet but also helps you make healthier choices, save time, and reduce food waste. As you integrate these tips into your routine, you'll find that meal planning becomes a valuable tool in achieving and maintaining your health and wellness goals.

Breakfast Choices

Breakfast Casserole

Cooking Time: 45 minutes Preparation Time: 20 minutes

Nutritional Info: Calories: 250 Protein: 18g Carbohydrates: 8g Fat: 16g

Serving: 6

INGREDIENTS:

- 8 eggs
- 2 cups spinach, chopped
- 1 cup bell peppers, diced
- 1/2 cup onion, chopped
- 1 cup turkey sausage, cooked and crumbled
- 1 cup cheese, shredded

INSTRUCTIONS:

1. Preheat the oven to 375°F (190°C).
2. In a skillet, cook turkey sausage until browned.
3. In a greased baking dish, layer spinach, bell peppers, onion, cooked sausage, and cheese.
4. In a bowl, whisk eggs and pour over the layers.
5. Bake for 40-45 minutes until eggs are set.
6. Let it cool slightly before slicing.

Kale and Spinach Smoothie

Cooking Time: 5 minutes Preparation Time: 10 minutes

Nutritional Info: (Per serving) Calories: 150 Protein: 7g

Carbohydrates: 25g Fat: 3g

Serving: 2

INGREDIENTS:

- 1 cup kale, stems removed
- 1 cup spinach
- 1 banana
- 1/2 cup Greek yogurt
- 1 cup almond milk

INSTRUCTIONS:

1. In a blender, combine kale, spinach, banana, Greek yogurt, and almond milk.
2. Blend until smooth.
3. Pour into glasses and serve immediately.
4. Serving: 2 servings

Strawberry and Yogurt Parfait

Preparation Time: 10 minutes Nutritional Info: Calories: 300 Protein: 15g Carbohydrates: 45g Fat: 8g

Serving: 1

INGREDIENTS:

- ➢ 2 cups Greek yogurt
- ➢ 1 cup fresh strawberries, sliced
- ➢ 1 cup granola
- ➢ Honey for drizzling

INSTRUCTIONS:

1. In a glass or bowl, start with a layer of Greek yogurt.
2. Add a layer of sliced strawberries.
3. Sprinkle a layer of granola over the strawberries.
4. Repeat the layers until the glass is filled.
5. Drizzle honey on top.
6. Repeat the process for additional parfaits.
7. Serve immediately and enjoy the delightful layers of flavor and texture.

Egg and Veggie Muffin Cups

Cooking Time: 20 minutes Preparation Time: 15 minutes

Nutritional Info: Calories: 180 Protein: 12g Carbohydrates: 5g Fat: 12g

Serving: 4

INGREDIENTS:

- ➢ 6 eggs
- ➢ 1 cup spinach, chopped
- ➢ 1/2 cup cherry tomatoes, diced
- ➢ 1/4 cup bell peppers, diced
- ➢ 1/4 cup feta cheese, crumbled

INSTRUCTIONS:

1. Preheat the oven to 350°F (175°C).
2. In a bowl, whisk eggs and add chopped spinach, diced cherry tomatoes, bell peppers, and feta cheese.
3. Pour the mixture into greased muffin cups, filling each about two-thirds full.
4. Bake for 15-20 minutes until eggs are set.
5. Allow them to cool slightly before removing from the muffin tin.
6. Serve warm and enjoy these portable and flavorful egg muffin cups.

Veggie Breakfast Burrito

Cooking Time: 15 minutes Preparation Time: 20 minutes

Nutritional Info: Calories: 320 Protein: 15g Carbohydrates: 40g Fat: 12g

Serving: 2

INGREDIENTS:

- 2 whole wheat tortillas
- eggs
- 1/2 cup black beans, drained and rinsed
- 1/4 cup bell peppers, diced
- 1/4 cup onion, diced
- 1 avocado, sliced
- Salsa for topping

INSTRUCTIONS:

1. In a pan, sauté diced bell peppers and onions until softened.
2. Scramble eggs in the pan with the cooked vegetables.
3. Warm the whole wheat tortillas.
4. Fill each tortilla with the scrambled egg mixture.
5. Top with black beans, sliced avocado, and salsa.
6. Roll up the burritos and serve warm.

Broccoli and Parmesan Cheese Omelet

Cooking Time: 10 minutes Preparation Time: 10 minutes

Nutritional Info: Calories: 250 Protein: 20g Carbohydrates: 5g Fat: 16g

Serving: 1 serving

INGREDIENTS:

- ➢ eggs
- ➢ 1 cup broccoli florets, steamed
- ➢ 1/4 cup Parmesan cheese, grated
- ➢ Salt and pepper to taste
- ➢ Olive oil for cooking

INSTRUCTIONS:

1. Steam broccoli until tender.
2. In a bowl, whisk eggs and season with salt and pepper.
3. Heat olive oil in a pan over medium heat.
4. Pour the whisked eggs into the pan and allow them to set slightly.
5. Add steamed broccoli and sprinkle Parmesan cheese over one half of the omelet.
6. Carefully fold the other half of the omelet over the filling.
7. Cook for another 2-3 minutes until the omelet is fully cooked.
8. Slide the omelet onto a plate and serve immediately.

Egg Salad Avocado Toast

Preparation Time: 15 minutes Nutritional Info: Calories: 280

Protein: 15g Carbohydrates: 20g Fat: 16g

Serving: 2

INGREDIENTS:

- eggs
- 2 avocados
- slices whole grain bread
- 1/4 cup Greek yogurt
- 1 tablespoon Dijon mustard
- Salt and pepper to taste

INSTRUCTIONS:

1. Boil the eggs until hard-cooked. Once cooled, peel and chop them into small pieces.
2. In a bowl, mash the avocados. Add Greek yogurt and Dijon mustard, mixing until smooth.
3. Toast the whole grain bread slices to your preference.
4. Spread the avocado mixture generously over each slice of toasted bread.
5. Evenly distribute the chopped eggs on top of the avocado spread.
6. Add salt and pepper to taste.
7. Serve the egg salad avocado toast immediately.

Quinoa Breakfast Bowl

Cooking Time: 15 minutes Preparation Time: 10 minutes

Nutritional Info: Calories: 350 Protein: 12g Carbohydrates: 50g Fat: 10g

Serving: 1

INGREDIENTS:

- ➤ 1 cup quinoa
- ➤ 2 cups almond milk
- ➤ 1 cup mixed berries (strawberries, raspberries, blueberries)
- ➤ 1/4 cup almonds, sliced
- ➤ Honey for drizzling

INSTRUCTIONS:

1. Rinse the quinoa under cold water.
2. In a saucepan, combine quinoa and almond milk. Bring to a boil, then reduce heat and simmer for 15 minutes or until quinoa is cooked and liquid is absorbed.
3. Fluff the quinoa with a fork and divide it into serving bowls.
4. Top with mixed berries and sliced almonds.
5. Drizzle honey over the bowl just before serving.
6. Enjoy your nutritious and flavorful quinoa breakfast bowl.

Quinoa Breakfast Bowl

Cooking Time: 15 minutes Preparation Time: 10 minutes

Nutritional Info: Calories: 350 Protein: 12g Carbohydrates: 50g Fat: 10g

Serving: 1

INGREDIENTS:

- ➢ 1 cup quinoa
- ➢ 2 cups almond milk
- ➢ 1 cup mixed berries (strawberries, blueberries, raspberries)
- ➢ 1/4 cup almonds, sliced
- ➢ Honey for drizzling

INSTRUCTIONS:

1. Rinse the quinoa under cold water.
2. In a saucepan, combine quinoa and almond milk. Bring to a boil, then reduce heat and simmer for 15 minutes or until quinoa is cooked and liquid is absorbed.
3. Fluff the quinoa with a fork and divide it into serving bowls.
4. Top with mixed berries and sliced almonds.
5. Drizzle honey over the bowl just before serving.
6. Enjoy your nutritious and flavorful quinoa breakfast bowl.

Avocado and Arugula Omelet

Cooking Time: 10 minutes Preparation Time: 5 minutes

Nutritional Info: Calories: 280 Protein: 15g Carbohydrates: 10g Fat: 20g

Serving: 1

INGREDIENTS:

- eggs
- 1/2 avocado, sliced
- Handful of arugula
- Salt and pepper to taste
- Olive oil

INSTRUCTIONS:

1. Crack the eggs into a bowl, season with salt and pepper, and whisk until thoroughly combined.
2. Heat a non-stick skillet over medium heat and add a splash of olive oil.
3. Pour the whisked eggs into the skillet and allow them to set slightly.
4. Place avocado slices and arugula on one half of the omelet.
5. Carefully fold the other half of the omelet over the filling, creating a half-moon shape.
6. Cook for another 2-3 minutes until the omelet is fully cooked.
7. Slide the omelet onto a plate and serve immediately.

Waffles with Feta and Smoked Salmon

Cooking Time: 15 minutes Preparation Time: 10 minutes

Nutritional Info: Calories: 320 Protein: 18g Carbohydrates: 30g Fat: 15g

Serving: 2

INGREDIENTS:

- ➢ Whole grain waffle mix
- ➢ Feta cheese, crumbled
- ➢ Smoked salmon slices
- ➢ Fresh dill for garnish

INSTRUCTIONS:

1. Prepare the whole grain waffle mix according to the package instructions.
2. Once the waffles are cooked, place them on a plate.
3. Crumble feta cheese over the warm waffles.
4. Top with smoked salmon slices.
5. Garnish with fresh dill.
6. Serve the waffles warm and enjoy this delightful combination of flavors.

Granola Breakfast Protein Balls

Preparation Time: 20 minutes

Nutritional Info: Calories: 150 Protein: 8g Carbohydrates: 15g Fat: 7g

Serving: 12 balls

INGREDIENTS:

- 1 cup granola
- 1/2 cup almond butter
- 1/4 cup honey
- 1/2 cup protein powder
- 1/4 cup dark chocolate chips

INSTRUCTIONS:

1. In a bowl, combine granola, almond butter, honey, protein powder, and dark chocolate chips.
2. Mix until well combined.
3. Take small portions and roll into bite-sized balls.
4. Place them on a tray lined with parchment paper.
5. Refrigerate for at least 30 minutes to firm up.
6. Enjoy these protein-packed granola balls as a quick and energizing breakfast or snack.

Chia Seed Pudding Parfait

Preparation Time: 5 minutes (plus overnight chilling)

Nutritional Info: Calories: 200 Protein: 6g Carbohydrates: 25g Fat: 8g

Serving: 2

INGREDIENTS:

- ➤ 1/4 cup chia seeds
- ➤ 1 cup almond milk
- ➤ 1 teaspoon vanilla extract
- ➤ 1 tablespoon maple syrup
- ➤ Mixed berries for layering
- ➤ Granola for topping

INSTRUCTIONS:

1. In a jar, mix chia seeds, almond milk, vanilla extract, and maple syrup.
2. Refrigerate overnight or for at least 4 hours until it forms a pudding-like consistency.
3. In serving glasses, layer the chia pudding with mixed berries.
4. Top with granola before serving.
5. Enjoy this nutritious and delicious chia seed pudding parfait.

Tuna and Olive Spinach Salad

Preparation Time: 15 minutes

Nutritional Info: Calories: 280 Protein: 25g Carbohydrates: 10g Fat: 15g

Serving: 2

INGREDIENTS:

- 2 cups fresh spinach
- 1 can tuna, drained
- 1/4 cup Kalamata olives, sliced
- Cherry tomatoes, halved
- Cucumber, sliced
- Feta cheese, crumbled
- Olive oil and lemon dressing

INSTRUCTIONS:

1. In a large bowl, combine fresh spinach, drained tuna, sliced olives, cherry tomatoes, cucumber, and crumbled feta cheese.
2. Drizzle olive oil and lemon dressing over the salad.
3. Toss gently to combine all ingredients.
4. Serve this refreshing tuna and olive spinach salad for a light and nutritious meal.

Cacao Berry Smoothie

Preparation Time: 10 minutes

Nutritional Info: Calories: 150 Protein: 4g Carbohydrates: 30g Fat: 3g

Serving: 2

INGREDIENTS:

- ➢ 1 cup mixed berries (strawberries, blueberries, raspberries)
- ➢ 1 banana
- ➢ 2 tablespoons cacao powder
- ➢ 1 cup almond milk
- ➢ Ice cubes

INSTRUCTIONS:

1. In a blender, combine mixed berries, banana, cacao powder, almond milk, and ice cubes.
2. Blend until smooth and creamy.
3. Pour into glasses and enjoy this indulgent yet healthy cacao berry smoothie.

Spinach and Feta Scrambled Egg Pitas

Cooking Time: 10 minutes Preparation Time: 10 minutes

Nutritional Info: Calories: 280 Protein: 18g Carbohydrates: 20g Fat: 14g

Serving: 2

INGREDIENTS:

- eggs
- 1 cup fresh spinach, chopped
- 1/2 cup feta cheese, crumbled
- Whole wheat pitas
- Olive oil
- Salt and pepper to taste

INSTRUCTIONS:

1. In a bowl, whisk eggs and season with salt and pepper.
2. Olive oil should be heated in a pan over medium heat.
3. Add chopped spinach to the pan and sauté until wilted.
4. Pour the whisked eggs over the spinach and scramble until cooked.
5. Stir in crumbled feta cheese.
6. Warm whole wheat pitas.
7. Spoon the egg, spinach, and feta mixture into the pitas.
8. Serve these flavorful and protein-packed scrambled egg pitas.

Lunch ideas

Roasted Vegetable Wrap

Cooking Time: 25 minutes

Preparation Time: 15 minutes

Nutritional Info: Calories: 300 Protein: 8g Carbohydrates: 40g Fat: 12g

Serving: 2

INGREDIENTS:

- Whole wheat wraps
- Assorted vegetables (bell peppers, zucchini, and cherry tomatoes)
- Olive oil
- Hummus
- Fresh herbs (basil, parsley)

INSTRUCTIONS:

1. Preheat the oven to 400°F (200°C).
2. Toss chopped vegetables in olive oil and roast for 20-25 minutes until tender.
3. Spread hummus on each whole wheat wrap.
4. Fill wraps with the roasted vegetables and sprinkle fresh herbs.
5. Roll up and serve these delicious and colorful roasted vegetable wraps.

Greek Salmon Salad

Cooking Time: 15 minutes Preparation Time: 10 minutes

Nutritional Info: Calories: 350Protein: 25gCarbohydrates: 15g Fat: 22g

Serving: 2

INGREDIENTS:

- ➢ Grilled or baked salmon fillets
- ➢ Mixed greens
- ➢ Cherry tomatoes, halved
- ➢ Cucumber, sliced
- ➢ Red onion, thinly sliced
- ➢ Feta cheese, crumbled
- ➢ Kalamata olives
- ➢ Greek salad dressing

INSTRUCTIONS:

1. Grill or bake salmon until fully cooked.
2. In a large bowl, combine mixed greens, cherry tomatoes, cucumber, red onion, feta cheese, and Kalamata olives.
3. Top with grilled salmon.
4. Drizzle Greek salad dressing over the salad.
5. Toss gently and serve this fresh and protein-packed Greek salmon salad.

Shrimp and Quinoa Stir-Fry

Cooking Time: 20 minutes Preparation Time: 15 minutes

Nutritional Info: Calories: 320 Protein: 20g Carbohydrates: 40g Fat: 8g

Serving: 2

INGREDIENTS:

- ➢ 1 cup quinoa
- ➢ 2 cups water
- ➢ Shrimp, peeled and deveined
- ➢ Mixed vegetables (bell peppers, broccoli, carrots)
- ➢ Soy sauce
- ➢ Sesame oil
- ➢ Garlic, minced

INSTRUCTIONS:

1. Cook quinoa in water according to package instructions.
2. In a wok or skillet, heat sesame oil and sauté minced garlic.
3. Add shrimp and stir-fry until cooked.
4. Add mixed vegetables and continue to stir-fry until tender.
5. Mix in cooked quinoa and soy sauce.
6. Stir until well combined and serve this flavorful shrimp and quinoa stir-fry.

Couscous and Chickpea Salad

Cooking Time: 15 minutes Preparation Time: 10 minutes

Nutritional Info: Calories: 280Protein: 12g Carbohydrates: 40g Fat: 8g

Serving: 2

INGREDIENTS:

- ➢ 1 cup couscous
- ➢ 1 can chickpeas, drained and rinsed
- ➢ Cherry tomatoes, halved
- ➢ Cucumber, diced
- ➢ Red onion, finely chopped
- ➢ Feta cheese, crumbled
- ➢ Fresh mint leaves, chopped
- ➢ Olive oil and lemon dressing

INSTRUCTIONS:

1. Cook couscous according to package instructions.
2. In a large bowl, combine cooked couscous, chickpeas, cherry tomatoes, cucumber, red onion, feta cheese, and chopped mint.
3. Drizzle olive oil and lemon dressing over the salad and toss gently.
4. Serve this vibrant couscous and chickpea salad as a refreshing side or main dish.

Teriyaki Tofu Rice

Cooking Time: 20 minutes Preparation Time: 15 minutes

Nutritional Info: Calories: 320 Protein: 15g Carbohydrates: 50g Fat: 8g

Serving: 2

INGREDIENTS:

- ➢ Firm tofu, cubed
- ➢ Brown rice, cooked
- ➢ Broccoli florets
- ➢ Carrots, sliced
- ➢ Teriyaki sauce
- ➢ Sesame seeds for garnish

INSTRUCTIONS:

1. Press tofu to remove excess water and cut it into cubes.
2. In a pan, sauté tofu until golden brown.
3. Add broccoli florets and sliced carrots, and stir-fry until vegetables are tender.
4. Pour teriyaki sauce over the tofu and vegetables.
5. Serve the teriyaki tofu and vegetables over cooked brown rice.
6. Garnish with sesame seeds and enjoy this savory teriyaki tofu rice bowl.

Avocado Chicken Salad

Cooking Time: 20 minutes Preparation Time: 15 minutes

Nutritional Info: Calories: 280 Protein: 25g Carbohydrates: 15g Fat: 15g

Serving: 2

INGREDIENTS:

- ➢ Cooked chicken breast, shredded
- ➢ Avocado, diced
- ➢ Cherry tomatoes, halved
- ➢ Red onion, finely chopped
- ➢ Fresh cilantro, chopped
- ➢ Lime juice
- ➢ Salt and pepper to taste

INSTRUCTIONS:

1. In a large bowl, combine shredded chicken, diced avocado, cherry tomatoes, red onion, and chopped cilantro.
2. Drizzle lime juice over the ingredients.
3. Add salt and pepper to taste.
4. Toss gently until well mixed.
5. Serve this creamy and zesty avocado chicken salad on its own or over a bed of greens.

Spicy Ramen Cup of Noodles

Cooking Time: 15 minutes Preparation Time: 10 minutes

Nutritional Info: Calories: 320 Protein: 12g Carbohydrates: 45g Fat: 10g

SERVING: 2

INGREDIENTS:

- Ramen noodles
- Vegetable broth
- Tofu, cubed
- Mixed vegetables (spinach, mushrooms, green onions)
- Soy sauce
- Sriracha sauce

INSTRUCTIONS:

1. Cook the ramen noodles according per the package instructions.
2. In a pot, heat vegetable broth and add tofu, mixed vegetables, soy sauce, and sriracha.
3. Simmer until tofu is heated through, and vegetables are tender.
4. Pour the spicy ramen broth over cooked noodles.
5. Serve this quick and flavorful spicy ramen cup of noodles.

Chicken Tuna Salad

Cooking Time: 15 minutes Preparation Time: 10 minutes

Nutritional Info: Calories: 280 Protein: 25g Carbohydrates: 15g Fat: 12g

Serving: 2

INGREDIENTS:

- Canned tuna, drained
- Cooked chicken breast, shredded
- Celery, finely chopped
- Red grapes, halved
- Greek yogurt
- Dijon mustard
- Lemon juice
- Salt and pepper to taste

INSTRUCTIONS:

1. In a bowl, combine drained tuna, shredded chicken, chopped celery, and halved red grapes.
2. In a separate bowl, mix Greek yogurt, Dijon mustard, and lemon juice to create the dressing.
3. Pour the dressing over the tuna and chicken mixture.
4. Season with salt and pepper to taste.
5. Gently toss until all ingredients are coated.
6. Serve this delightful chicken tuna salad on a bed of greens or in a wrap.

Sweet Potato and Lentil Stew

Cooking Time: 30 minutes Preparation Time: 15 minutes

Nutritional Info: Calories: 300 Protein: 15g Carbohydrates: 50g Fat: 8g

Serving: 2

INGREDIENTS:

- ➢ Sweet potatoes, peeled and diced
- ➢ Lentils, rinsed
- ➢ Onion, diced
- ➢ Garlic, minced
- ➢ Vegetable broth
- ➢ Cumin, paprika, and cinnamon
- ➢ Coconut milk
- ➢ Fresh cilantro for garnish

INSTRUCTIONS:

1. In a pot, sauté diced onion and minced garlic until softened.
2. Add sweet potatoes, lentils, vegetable broth, cumin, paprika, and cinnamon to the pot.
3. Simmer until sweet potatoes and lentils are tender.
4. Stir in coconut milk for creaminess.
5. Garnish with fresh cilantro before serving this hearty sweet potato and lentil stew.

Turmeric Chicken Wrap

Cooking Time: 20 minutes Preparation Time: 15 minutes

Nutritional Info: Calories: 320 Protein: 25g Carbohydrates: 30g Fat: 12g

Serving: 2

INGREDIENTS:

- ➢ Chicken breast, sliced
- ➢ Turmeric powder
- ➢ Whole wheat wraps
- ➢ Greek yogurt
- ➢ Cucumber, thinly sliced
- ➢ Red onion, thinly sliced
- ➢ Fresh mint leaves

INSTRUCTIONS:

1. Season sliced chicken breast with turmeric powder and cook until fully cooked.
2. Warm whole wheat wraps in a pan or microwave.
3. Spread Greek yogurt on each wrap.
4. Place cooked turmeric chicken slices, cucumber, red onion, and fresh mint leaves on the wraps.
5. Roll up the wraps and secure with toothpicks if needed.
6. Enjoy these flavorful and vibrant turmeric chicken wraps.

Dinner Recipes

Eggplant Rollatini with Tomato Sauce

Cooking Time: 45 minutes Preparation Time: 20 minutes

Nutritional Info: Calories: 280 Protein: 15g Carbohydrates: 20g Fat: 16g

Serving: 4

INGREDIENTS:

- ➢ Eggplants, thinly sliced
- ➢ Ricotta cheese
- ➢ Spinach, chopped
- ➢ Parmesan cheese
- ➢ Marinara sauce
- ➢ Mozzarella cheese

INSTRUCTIONS:

1. Preheat the oven to 375°F (190°C).
2. Mix ricotta cheese with chopped spinach and Parmesan.
3. Place a spoonful of the ricotta mixture onto each eggplant slice and roll up.
4. Arrange the rolled eggplants in a baking dish, cover with marinara sauce, and sprinkle with mozzarella.
5. Bake until the cheese is melts and bubbles.
6. Serve this delicious eggplant rollatini with tomato sauce.

Lemon Dill Baked Cod:

Cooking Time: 20 minutes Preparation Time: 15 minutes

Nutritional Info: Calories: 220 Protein: 25g Carbohydrates: 2g Fat: 12g

Serving: 2

INGREDIENTS:

- Cod fillets
- Lemon, sliced
- Fresh dill, chopped
- Garlic, minced
- Olive oil

INSTRUCTIONS:

1. Preheat the oven to 400°F (200°C).
2. Place cod fillets on a baking sheet.
3. Drizzle with olive oil, sprinkle minced garlic, and top with lemon slices and chopped dill.
4. Bake until the cod is cooked through.
5. Serve this light and flavorful lemon dill baked cod.

Buffalo Cauliflower Tacos

Cooking Time: 25 minutes Preparation Time: 15 minutes

Nutritional Info: Calories: 280 Protein: 5g Carbohydrates: 30g Fat: 16g

Serving: 4

INGREDIENTS:

- ➢ Cauliflower florets
- ➢ Buffalo sauce
- ➢ Corn tortillas
- ➢ Cabbage, shredded
- ➢ Avocado, sliced
- ➢ Ranch dressing

INSTRUCTIONS:

1. Toss cauliflower florets in buffalo sauce and bake until crispy.
2. Warm corn tortillas.
3. Fill tortillas with buffalo cauliflower, shredded cabbage, and sliced avocado.
4. Drizzle with ranch dressing.
5. Serve these spicy and flavorful buffalo cauliflower tacos.

Chicken Cali Soup

Cooking Time: 30 minutes Preparation Time: 20 minutes

Nutritional Info: Calories: 320 Protein: 25g Carbohydrates: 15g Fat: 18g

Serving: 4

INGREDIENTS:

- Chicken breasts, cooked and shredded
- Cauliflower rice
- Bell peppers, diced
- Avocado, sliced
- Lime juice
- Cilantro, chopped

INSTRUCTIONS:

1. In a pot, combine shredded chicken, cauliflower rice, and diced bell peppers.
2. Simmer until the vegetables are tender.
3. Ladle the soup into bowls and top with sliced avocado, lime juice, and chopped cilantro.
4. Serve this hearty and nutritious chicken Cali soup.

Butternut Squash and Sage Risotto

Cooking Time: 40 minutes Preparation Time: 15 minutes

Nutritional Info: Calories: 300 Protein: 8g Carbohydrates: 60g Fat: 4g

Serving: 4 Servings

INGREDIENTS:

- ➢ Arborio rice
- ➢ Butternut squash, diced
- ➢ Vegetable broth
- ➢ Onion, finely chopped
- ➢ Fresh sage leaves
- ➢ Parmesan cheese, grated

INSTRUCTIONS:

1. In a pan, sauté chopped onion until translucent.
2. Add Arborio rice and stir until lightly toasted.
3. Gradually add vegetable broth, stirring continuously until absorbed.
4. Stir in diced butternut squash and fresh sage leaves.
5. Continue adding broth until the rice is creamy and cooked.
6. Finish with grated Parmesan cheese.
7. Serve this comforting butternut squash and sage risotto.

Cauliflower Steak with Pesto

Cooking Time: 30 minutes Preparation Time: 15 minutes

Nutritional Info: Calories: 250 Protein: 8g Carbohydrates: 20g Fat: 18g

Serving: 2

INGREDIENTS:

- ➢ Cauliflower, sliced into steaks
- ➢ Pesto sauce
- ➢ Cherry tomatoes, halved
- ➢ Pine nuts, toasted
- ➢ Fresh basil leaves

INSTRUCTIONS:

1. Brush cauliflower steaks with pesto sauce.
2. Roast or grill until cauliflower is tender.
3. Arrange on a plate and top with halved cherry tomatoes.
4. Sprinkle with toasted pine nuts and fresh basil leaves.
5. Serve this elegant cauliflower steak with pesto.

Vegetarian Stuffed Bell Peppers

Cooking Time: 45 minutes Preparation Time: 20 minutes

Nutritional Info: Calories: 280 Protein: 12g Carbohydrates: 40g Fat: 8g

Serving: 4

INGREDIENTS:

- ➢ Bell peppers, halved and cleaned
- ➢ Quinoa, cooked
- ➢ Black beans, drained and rinsed
- ➢ Corn kernels
- ➢ Salsa
- ➢ Cumin, chili powder, and garlic powder
- ➢ Shredded cheese

INSTRUCTIONS:

1. Preheat the oven to 375°F (190°C).
2. In a bowl, mix cooked quinoa, black beans, corn, salsa, and spices.
3. Stuff bell pepper halves with the quinoa mixture.
4. Top with shredded cheese.
5. Bake until peppers are tender and cheese is melted.
6. Serve these flavorful and nutritious vegetarian stuffed bell peppers.

Portobello Mushroom Bell

Cooking Time: 25 minutes Preparation Time: 15 minutes

Nutritional Info: Calories: 250 Protein: 15g Carbohydrates: 30g Fat: 10g

Serving: 2

INGREDIENTS:

- ➢ Portobello mushrooms, stems removed
- ➢ Quinoa, cooked
- ➢ Spinach, sautéed
- ➢ Feta cheese, crumbled
- ➢ Balsamic glaze

INSTRUCTIONS:

1. Preheat the oven to 400°F (200°C).
2. Place Portobello mushrooms on a baking sheet.
3. Fill each mushroom with cooked quinoa, sautéed spinach, and crumbled feta.
4. Bake until mushrooms are tender.
5. Drizzle with balsamic glaze before serving.
6. Enjoy this savory and satisfying portobello mushroom bell.

Minestra Maritata

Cooking Time: 40 minutes Preparation Time: 20 minutes

Nutritional Info: Calories: 320 Protein: 18g Carbohydrates: 25g Fat: 16g

Serving: 4

INGREDIENTS:

- Italian sausage, sliced
- Kale, chopped
- Cannellini beans, cooked
- Carrots, diced
- Celery, sliced
- Chicken broth
- Garlic, minced

INSTRUCTIONS:

1. In a pot, sauté sliced Italian sausage until browned.
2. Add the minced garlic and cook until fragrant.
3. Stir in chopped kale, diced carrots, sliced celery, and cooked cannellini beans.
4. Pour in chicken broth and simmer until vegetables are tender.
5. Serve this hearty and flavorful minestra maritata.

Sheet Pan Shrimp and Beets

Cooking Time: 30 minutes Preparation Time: 15 minutes

Nutritional Info: Calories: 280 Protein: 20g Carbohydrates: 20g Fat: 14g

Serving: 2

INGREDIENTS:

- Shrimp, peeled and deveined
- Beets, peeled and sliced
- Olive oil
- Garlic powder, paprika, salt, and pepper
- Fresh parsley, chopped

INSTRUCTIONS:

1. Preheat the oven to 400°F (200°C).
2. Toss shrimp and sliced beets with olive oil, garlic powder, paprika, salt, and pepper on a sheet pan.
3. Roast until shrimp are pink and beets are tender.
4. Garnish with fresh chopped parsley before serving.
5. Enjoy this easy and delicious sheet pan shrimp and beets.

Snack Recipes

Avocado Hummus

Preparation Time: 10 minutes

Nutritional Info: Calories: 180 Protein: 6g Carbohydrates: 15g Fat: 10g

Serving: 4

INGREDIENTS:

- Chickpeas, drained and rinsed
- Avocado
- Tahini
- Lemon juice
- Garlic, minced
- Olive oil

INSTRUCTIONS:

1. In a food processor, blend chickpeas, avocado, tahini, lemon juice, and minced garlic until smooth.
2. Drizzle olive oil while blending until desired consistency is reached.
3. Serve this creamy and nutritious avocado hummus.

Trail Mix with Nuts and Seeds

Preparation Time: 5 minutes

Nutritional Info: Calories: 200 Protein: 5g Carbohydrates: 15g Fat: 14g

Serving: 4

INGREDIENTS:

- Almonds
- Walnuts
- Pumpkin seeds
- Sunflower seeds
- Dried cranberries
- Dark chocolate chips

INSTRUCTIONS:

1. Mix almonds, walnuts, pumpkin seeds, sunflower seeds, dried cranberries, and dark chocolate chips in a bowl.
2. Portion into snack-sized servings.
3. Enjoy this energizing trail mix with nuts and seeds.

Zucchini Pizza Bites

Cooking Time: 15 minutes Preparation Time: 10 minutes

Nutritional Info: Calories: 120 Protein: 6Carbohydrates: 10g Fat: 7g

Serving: 4

INGREDIENTS:

- ➢ Zucchini, sliced
- ➢ Tomato sauce
- ➢ Mozzarella cheese, shredded
- ➢ Cherry tomatoes, halved
- ➢ Fresh basil leaves

INSTRUCTIONS:

1. Preheat the oven to 375°F (190°C).
2. Place the zucchini slices on a baking sheet.
3. Top each slice with tomato sauce, shredded mozzarella, and a halved cherry tomato.
4. Bake until the cheese is melted and bubbly.
5. Garnish with fresh basil leaves.
6. Serve these delightful zucchini pizza bites.

Edamame and Sea Salt

Cooking Time: 5 minutes Preparation Time: 5 minutes

Nutritional Info: Calories: 90Protein: 8gCarbohydrates: 8g Fat: 4g

Serving: 4

INGREDIENTS:

- Edamame, steamed
- Sea salt

INSTRUCTIONS:

1. Steam edamame according to package instructions.
2. Sprinkle with sea salt.
3. Serve this simple and nutritious edamame with sea salt.

Peanut Butter Oat Energy Balls

Preparation Time: 15 minutes

Nutritional Info: Calories: 180 Protein: 5g Carbohydrates: 15g Fat: 10g

Serving: 4

INGREDIENTS:

- ➢ Rolled oats
- ➢ Peanut butter
- ➢ Honey
- ➢ Chia seeds
- ➢ Dark chocolate chips

INSTRUCTIONS:

1. In a bowl, mix rolled oats, peanut butter, honey, chia seeds, and dark chocolate chips.
2. Roll the mixture into bite-sized energy balls.
3. Refrigerate for at least 30 minutes.
4. Enjoy these delicious and energizing peanut butter oat energy balls.

Cucumber Avocado Roll-Up

Preparation Time: 10 minutes

Nutritional Info: Calories: 90 Protein: 2g Carbohydrates: 8g Fat: 6g

Serving: 4

INGREDIENTS:

- ➤ Cucumber, thinly sliced
- ➤ Avocado
- ➤ Hummus
- ➤ Cherry tomatoes, sliced

INSTRUCTIONS:

1. Lay cucumber slices flat.
2. Spread hummus on each slice.
3. Add a slice of avocado and a few cherry tomato slices.
4. Roll up and secure with toothpicks if needed.
5. Enjoy these refreshing cucumber avocado roll-ups.

Mango Date Energy Bites

Preparation Time: 15 minutes

Nutritional Info: Calories: 150 Protein: 3g Carbohydrates: 20g Fat: 7g

Serving: 4

INGREDIENTS:

- Dried mango, chopped
- Dates, pitted
- Almonds
- Coconut flakes
- Vanilla extract

INSTRUCTIONS:

1. In a food processor, blend dried mango, pitted dates, almonds, coconut flakes, and vanilla extract until a sticky mixture forms.
2. Roll the mixture into small energy bites.
3. Refrigerate for at least 20 minutes.
4. Indulge in these tropical-flavored mango date energy bites.

Carrot and Hummus Dippers

Preparation Time: 10 minutes

Nutritional Info: Calories: 60 Protein: 2g Carbohydrates: 10g Fat: 2g

Serving: 4

INGREDIENTS:

- ➤ Carrot sticks
- ➤ Hummus

INSTRUCTIONS:

1. Arrange carrot sticks on a plate.
2. Serve with hummus for dipping.
3. Enjoy this crunchy and satisfying carrot and hummus snack.

Almond Butter Energy Bites

Preparation Time: 15 minutes

Nutritional Info: Calories: 160 Protein: 5g Carbohydrates: 15g Fat: 10g

Serving: 4

INGREDIENTS:

- ➢ Almond butter
- ➢ Rolled oats
- ➢ Honey
- ➢ Flaxseeds, ground
- ➢ Dark chocolate chips

INSTRUCTIONS:

1. In a bowl, mix almond butter, rolled oats, honey, ground flaxseeds, and dark chocolate chips.
2. Form the mixture into bite-sized energy bites.
3. Refrigerate for at least 30 minutes.
4. Savor these nutritious and satisfying almond butter energy bites.

Garlic Hummus

Preparation Time: 10 minutes

Nutritional Info: Calories: 100 Protein: 4g Carbohydrates: 10g Fat: 6g

Serving: 4

INGREDIENTS:

- Chickpeas, drained and rinsed
- Garlic cloves
- Tahini
- Lemon juice
- Olive oil

INSTRUCTIONS:

1. In a food processor, blend chickpeas, garlic cloves, tahini, and lemon juice until smooth.
2. Drizzle olive oil while blending until desired consistency is reached.
3. Serve this flavorful and garlicky hummus.

Desert Recipes

Apple Chips

Cooking Time: 2 hours Preparation Time: 15 minutes

Nutritional Info: Calories: 50 Carbohydrates: 14g

Serving: 4

INGREDIENTS:

- ➢ Apples, thinly sliced
- ➢ Cinnamon
- ➢ Sugar (optional)

INSTRUCTIONS:

1. Preheat oven to 200°F (93°C).
2. Arrange thinly sliced apples on a baking sheet.
3. Sprinkle with cinnamon and sugar if desired.
4. Bake until the edges are crisp.
5. Allow to cool before enjoying these crunchy apple chips

Peach and Mint Sorbet

Preparation Time: 10 minutes

Nutritional Info: Calories: 70 Protein: 1g Carbohydrates: 18g

Serving: 4 servings

INGREDIENTS:

- ➤ Peaches, peeled and sliced
- ➤ Fresh mint leaves
- ➤ Lemon juice
- ➤ Honey (optional)

INSTRUCTIONS:

1. Blend sliced peaches, mint leaves, lemon juice, and honey until smooth.
2. Pour the mixture into a shallow dish and freeze.
3. Stir every 30 minutes until set.
4. Serve this refreshing peach and mint sorbet.

Turmeric Ginger Cookies

Cooking Time: 12 minutes Preparation Time: 15 minutes

Nutritional Info: Calories: 180 Protein: 2g Carbohydrates: 25g Fat: 8g

Serving: 4

INGREDIENTS:

- ➢ All-purpose flour
- ➢ Turmeric powder
- ➢ Ground ginger
- ➢ Butter, softened
- ➢ Brown sugar
- ➢ Egg

INSTRUCTIONS:

1. Preheat oven to 350°F (175°C).
2. In a bowl, whisk together flour, turmeric powder, and ground ginger.
3. In another bowl, cream together softened butter and brown sugar.
4. Add an egg to the butter-sugar mixture and mix well.
5. Gradually incorporate the dry ingredients.
6. Scoop dough onto a baking sheet and bake until edges are golden.
7. Allow to cool before enjoying these spiced turmeric ginger cookies.

Mango Coconut Ice Cream

Preparation Time: 10 minutes

Nutritional Info: Calories: 120 Protein: 1g Carbohydrates: 25g Fat: 2g

Serving: 4

INGREDIENTS:

- ➢ Mango, frozen
- ➢ Coconut milk
- ➢ Maple syrup (optional)

INSTRUCTIONS:

1. Blend frozen mango and coconut milk until smooth.
2. If you want sweetness add maple syrup.
3. Freeze until set or enjoy immediately as soft-serve.
4. Scoop and relish this tropical mango coconut ice cream.

Chocolate Dipped Frozen Banana

Preparation Time: 10 minutes

Nutritional Info: Calories: 150 Protein: 2g Carbohydrates: 25g Fat: 6g

Serving: 4

INGREDIENTS:

- Bananas, peeled and halved
- Dark chocolate, melted
- Nuts or coconut flakes (optional)

INSTRUCTIONS:

1. Insert Popsicle sticks into banana halves.
2. Dip each banana into melted dark chocolate.
3. Optionally, coat with nuts or coconut flakes.
4. Place on a tray and freeze until the chocolate is set.
5. Indulge in these delightful chocolate-dipped frozen bananas.

Mixed Berry Crisp

Cooking Time: 30 minutes Preparation Time: 15 minutes

Nutritional Info: Calories: 200 Protein: 3g Carbohydrates: 30g Fat: 8g

Serving: 4

INGREDIENTS:

- Mixed berries (strawberries, blueberries, raspberries)
- Rolled oats
- Almond flour
- Maple syrup
- Coconut oil

INSTRUCTIONS:

1. Preheat oven to 350°F (175°C).
2. Toss mixed berries with maple syrup and place in a baking dish.
3. In a bowl, mix rolled oats, almond flour, and melted coconut oil.
4. The oat mixture should be spread over the berries.
5. Bake until the top is golden and the berries are bubbling.
6. Serve warm, savoring the delicious mixed berry crisp.

Long-Term Success and Lifestyle Tips

Maintaining Consistency

Overcoming Challenges

Embarking on the journey of adopting an anti-inflammatory diet for beginners may present certain challenges, but with awareness and proactive strategies, these obstacles can be effectively overcome. **Here are some common challenges and tips to conquer them:**

1. **Lack of Knowledge:**
   - **Challenge:** Understanding the principles of an anti-inflammatory diet can be overwhelming for beginners.
   - **Solution:** Educate yourself through reliable sources, consult with nutritionists, and gradually integrate new information into your daily routine.
2. **Taste Preferences:**
   - **Challenge:** Adapting to new flavors and ingredients can be challenging, especially if you have been accustomed to a different taste profile.
   - **Solution:** Experiment with herbs, spices, and alternative cooking methods to enhance flavors. Gradually introduce new ingredients to allow your taste buds to adjust.
3. **Time Constraints:**
   - **Challenge:** Busy schedules may pose a barrier to preparing fresh and wholesome meals.
   - **Solution:** Plan and prep meals in advance, utilize batch cooking, and explore quick and simple recipes. Prioritize your health by allocating time for meal preparation.

4. Social Pressures:
   - ➤ **Challenge:** Navigating social situations where dietary choices may differ can be uncomfortable.
   - ➤ **Solution:** Communicate your dietary preferences politely, bring your own dishes to gatherings, and focus on the social aspect rather than solely on the food.
5. **Availability of Ingredients:**
   - ➤ **Challenge:** Locating specific anti-inflammatory ingredients may be challenging, depending on your location.
   - ➤ **Solution:** Explore local markets, health food stores, and online options. Consider alternatives if certain ingredients are not readily available.
6. **Emotional Eating:**
   - ➤ **Challenge:** Emotional triggers leading to unhealthy food choices can hinder progress.
   - ➤ **Solution:** Practice mindfulness, identify emotional triggers, and seek alternative coping mechanisms such as exercise, meditation, or seeking support from friends and family.
7. **Sustainability:**
   - ➤ **Challenge:** Maintaining a long-term commitment to an anti-inflammatory lifestyle.
   - ➤ **Solution:** Set realistic goals, focus on gradual changes, and celebrate small victories. Connect with a supportive community for encouragement and inspiration.

Remember that transitioning to an anti-inflammatory diet is a personal journey, and overcoming challenges involves persistence, self-compassion, and a commitment to long-term well-being.

Conclusion

In conclusion, adopting an anti-inflammatory diet for beginners is a transformative journey towards enhancing your health and well-being. By prioritizing nutrient-rich foods, reducing inflammation, and making mindful dietary choices, you have taken proactive steps towards optimizing your overall health.

Throughout this process, you have learned about the basics of inflammation, the impact of chronic inflammation on health, and the numerous benefits of embracing an anti-inflammatory diet. Armed with knowledge, you have overcome challenges, stayed motivated, and made positive changes to your lifestyle.

As you continue on this path, remember to set clear goals, diversify your menu, track your progress, and prioritize self-care. Building a strong support system and celebrating achievements along the way will further fuel your motivation and commitment to long-term health.

Thank you for choosing "The Complete Anti-Inflammatory Diet Cookbook for Beginners." We sincerely hope that the recipes, guidance, and information provided in this cookbook have empowered you to embark on a journey towards better health and vitality.

Wishing you continued success and well-being on your anti-inflammatory diet journey.

Warm regards,

Vanessa R. Haddock

I have a request

Dear Valued Reader,

I hope you've enjoyed exploring the delectable world of "THE COMPLETE ANTI-INFLAMMATORY DIET COOKBOOK FOR BEGINNERS" as much as i enjoyed creating it. Your feedback means the world to me, and i would love to hear about your experiences with the recipes, your favorite dishes, and any creative twists you added to make them your own.

If this cookbook has added a dash of flavor, health, or joy to your kitchen, i invite you to share your thoughts by leaving a review. Your insights can inspire others to embark on their own culinary adventures and embrace the vibrant and nourishing Anti-inflammatory lifestyle.

To leave a review, simply visit the platform where you purchased or discovered this book, whether it's an online retailer, a book review website. Your feedback not only helps me improve but also contributes to building a community of passionate home cooks.

Thank you for being a part of this journey. Your reviews are the secret ingredient that makes my cookbook experience even more special.

Happy cooking, and i can't wait to read your reviews.

Warm regards,

[Vanessa R. Haddock]

Additional Resources

Dear Esteemed Reader,

If "The complete Anti-Inflammatory Diet cookbook for Beginners" resonated with you, I believe you'll find more value in my other works. Explore a range of topics designed to enhance your well-being and knowledge. Visit my author page for a curated collection of books that aim to inspire, inform, and accompany you on various aspects of your journey.

To explore these books and more, please visit my Author central page on Amazon. There you will find a complete collection of my works that may pique your interest.

You can scan the QR code below or click the link to visit my Author central.

https://www.amazon.com/author/vanehad.com

Thank you for your continued support, and I look forward to being a part of your ongoing literary exploration.

Best Wishes,

Vanessa R. Haddock